The Boiled Egg Diet
The Easy, Fast Way to Weight Loss!

and is universal as so. The presentation of the information is without contract or any type of guarantee assurance.

The trademarks that are used are without any consent, and the publication of the trademark is without permission or backing by the trademark owner. All trademarks and brands within this book are for clarifying purposes only and are the owned by the owners themselves, not affiliated with this document.

Sign Up for Recipes, Tips and Tricks and more at:

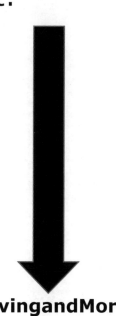

HealthyLivingandMore.com

Table of Contents

Introduction 15

    The Traditional Diet 15

    Egg & Grapefruit Version 17

    Egg Only Diet 17

    Some Pros & Cons 18

        Pros: 18

        Cons: 19

Benefits of Eggs 23

    Loaded with Nutrients 23

    Quality Protein 23

    Healthy Eyes 24

    Steady Blood Sugar 25

    A Healthy Brain 26

    Weight Loss 26

    Strengthen Nails, Hair & Bones 27

Some FAQ 29

    So what are some recommended
    foods? 29

Do I need to exercise with this diet? 30

Is the hardboiled egg diet considered to be expensive?..............31

Can you consume any fats on this diet?..32

Can I have any sweetener?...............32

Will I suffer from constipation?........33

Will I suffer from digestive issues on this diet? 33

Will I gain the weight back?..............34

How to Boil an Egg 35

Step 1: Get Your Eggs Started 35

Step 2: Start the Boil...........................36

Step 3: Let Your Eggs Sit...................36

Step 4: Use an Ice Bath 37

Recipes to Get You Started 39

Eggs on a Bed...40

Onion Skin Eggs.......................................41

Salmon Deviled Eggs 43

Egg & Asparagus Salad.......................46

Spinach & Egg Salad.............................48

Creamed Eggs 50

Teriyaki Eggs...52

Polished Eggs 54

Buffalo Ranch Deviled Eggs..............56

Simple Salad 58

Chesapeake Deviled Eggs 60

Pickled Eggs...62

Avocado Egg Salad 64

Cauliflower Egg Salad 65

Egg Guacamole 67

Tuna Salad 68

Egg Kulambu...69

Wasabi Deviled Eggs............................72

Egg Curry 74

Bacon Jalapeno Deviled Eggs...........76

Dill Pickle Deviled Eggs 78

Special Bacon Blue Eggs.....................80

Egg Chaat...84

Lean Scotch Eggs 86

Spicy Egg Salad Celery 89

Salad Recipes..93

Steak Salad...94

Cucumber & Tomato Salad................96

Cobb Salad...98

Cucumber & Dill Salad.......................100

Green Bean Salad 101

Balsamic Beet Salad...........................103

Massaged Kale Salad 105

Grilled Romaine Lettuce Salad.......105

Watermelon & Feta Salad 108

More Vegetable Pairings......................111

Roasted Bok Choy 112

Roasted Cabbage.................................114

Grilled Baby Bok Choy.......................116

Grilled Asparagus 117

Steamed Broccoli.................................119

Sautéed Kale...121

Mustard Greens & Onion 123

Boiled Cabbage 125

Lean Meats to Add In............................127

Skinless Poultry....................................127

Lean Beef..128

Lamb & Pork 129

Fish 129

Keeping Your Meat Lean 130

What about Bacon? 130

Lean Meat Recipes 133

Lemon Grilled Salmon 134

Easy Baked Chicken 136

Lemon & Basil Pork Chops 138

Baked Pork Chop 140

Grilled Greek Lemon Chicken 142

Grilled Blackened Tuna 144

Cajun Baked Salmon 146

Broiled Flounder with Lemon Butter
.... 148

Rosemary & Garlic Grilled Lamb 150

Grilled Sirloin 152

Lemon Pepper Tilapia 154

Different Types of Eggs 157

Brown Eggs vs. White Eggs 157

Duck Eggs vs. Chicken Eggs 158

Organic 160

Omega-3 Enriched 162

Vegetarian Fed 162

Check the Grade of Egg....................163

One Week Meal Plan..............................165

Sunday 165

Monday 166

Tuesday..166

Wednesday 166

Thursday...167

Friday 167

Saturday 168

Some Fruit Variety..................................169

Lemons & Limes...................................169

Blood Oranges 170

Grapefruit 170

Oranges...171

Watermelon 171

Strawberries...172

Cantaloupe...172

Peaches 173

Some Extra Tips......................................175

Get Your Fiber......................................175

Keep Hydrated!...................................176

Avoid Alcohol & Junk Food...............176

Get Some Sleep..................................177

Conclusion...179

Introduction

The Egg Diet has become popular because it'll help you successfully lose weight in a short amount of time by only eating eggs! Many celebrities have used it, including Charles Saatchi, Nigella Lawson's husband, reportedly lost over sixty pounds eating eggs for ten months he apparently ate an egg nine times a day. What most people don't know is that there are several versions of the Hard Boiled egg diet out there, so let's take a look at the three most popular versions and break them down.

The Traditional Diet

The most popular version is the traditional version, but you don't actually have to eat only eggs when you're using this version. However, you will get the majority of the protein you need from eggs its' a variation of the Atkins diet, and you'll focus on restricting the amount of carbs that you take in.

For the traditional diet, you need to eat two or more eggs for breakfast along with a low carb vegetable and a piece of fruit. Instead of a low carb vegetable you are also allowed to eat a lean protein. Lunch would be another serving of eggs or a lean, but small amount of protein. This usually includes fish or chicken. Dinner will also include more eggs or a lean protein such as chicken or fish. In this version of the diet, you're able to have low carbs vegetables and salads as desired. Fruits are limited to one or two servings a day, and carbs are strictly limited. This means almost no potatoes, pasta or bread.

Egg & Grapefruit Version

Another version of the diet is called the Egg and Grapefruit diet, which includes eating a half a grapefruit with each meal. Other than that, it's similar to the traditional diet. It's thought that the grapefruit will speed up weight loss, but there's less freedom in this diet. That's the reason this version doesn't work well for most people.

Egg Only Diet

This is the extreme version of the diet, so it doesn't work well for most people. This version is where you'll only eat hard boiled eggs and drink water or a crystal light drink mix for each and every meal. You'll grow tired of hardboiled eggs quickly, but you also run the risk of become malnourished and suffering from unhealthy bowel

function because eggs have zero
fiber.

Some Pros & Cons

In this book we'll mostly be looking
at the traditional boiled egg diet.
Here are some pros and cons to
consider.

Pros:

- **Reduced Appetite:** A high
  protein diet that consists of
  low carbs is known to reduce
  your appetite so you feel less
  hungry despite dieting
- **Increased Calorie Burn:**
  Since you're dealing with
  higher protein, you're going
  to be burn calories quicker
- **Vitamins:** Not only are eggs
  a good source of protein, but
  they're a good source of
  vitamins too.

- **Weight Loss:** This one probably comes without saying. Eating eggs, especially for breakfast, is known to increase your weight loss

Cons:

- **Not Balanced:** This is not a balanced approach to eaten since it eliminates entire food groups, including many vegetables.
- **Difficult Exercise:** With a lack of carbs it can be difficult, especially at first, to do any strenuous activity. Though, with this diet you don't need extensive exercise to lose the weight you want.
- **Fatigue & Nausea:** Many people deal with nausea and fatigue for a few days in the beginning. Your body has to adapt to the lowered intake of carbs.

- **Boredom:** Since you're eating the same day in and day out, it can be easy to get bored on the diet, making it hard to stick to.

Luckily, if you're determined you can still use this diet for real weight loss! The best part is that you'll see results quickly.

Chapter 1: Benefits of Eggs

Now that you know what the hardboiled egg diet is, let's explore some of the healthy benefits to adding eggs to your diet!

Loaded with Nutrients

Eggs contain many important vitamins and minerals such as vitamin A, D, B-6, and B-12. It also contains calcium, magnesium, and even iron. A single boiled egg can contain ten percent of your daily vitamin B-12, A, B-6, B-3, and vitamin D. It also contains two percent of your iron and calcium.

Quality Protein

You'll find that chicken eggs have over six grams of protein for each egg, which makes them a great choice for bodybuilders too! Don't worry though, the hardboiled egg diet will not bulk you up! It takes about thirty grams of meat to equal the same protein you get from a single egg, making it a higher quality protein choice. The protein is also rated higher than the protein you get from chicken or beef, and the coast of the egg versus the cost of the chicken or beef makes it much more affordable too.

Healthy Eyes

Your eyes will diminish over time, which is often referred to as macular degeneration, which can also occur simply due to age. This can lead to blindness. Eyes actually have two key nutrients to protect your eyes though which are lutein and zeaxanthin. These nutrients can also help to protect them from dangerous light wavelengths too if you're worried about your eyesight, then eggs are a great addition to your diet.

Steady Blood Sugar

The protein as well as the fat in your eggs will help to keep your blood sugar levels steady. This can help to prevent complications if you're diabetic since those complications result in higher blood sugar levels. Keep in mind that despite reports saying that eggs can raise cholesterol if you're diabetic, this isn't true if you're sticking to a low carb diet. With a low carb diet, eggs can actually help to decrease your cholesterol as a whole over time. In turn, this can help to decrease the risk of heart disease, especially when you add in their weight loss benefits.

A Healthy Brain

Choline is a nutrient that's essential for your brain's health. It aids in memory unction as well as brain growth. It's critical for women who are pregnant too since a growing baby will leave a mother's levels critically low. It's estimated that as much as ninety percent of people actually have low levels of choline. Therefore, by consuming eggs you're actually doing your brain a favor by providing it with a nutrient it desperately needs.

Weight Loss

If you're looking at the hardboiled egg diet, you already know that eggs can help to aid in weight loss. They can help to battle hunger too. They increase your feeling of fullness, allowing you to feel fuller for longer. This will help you to get through the day without those pesky hunger pangs getting in your way, especially when you're trying to trim down.

Strengthen Nails, Hair & Bones

Eggs are especially helpful if you can't eat dairy products, since they'll boost your vitamin D as well as your calcium levels. These can even help to prevent osteoporosis. Omega-3 fatty acids are also found in eggs, which will help to strengthen your hair, nails and bones.

Chapter 2: Some FAQ

Before you get started, you'll need to go through the common FAQ surrounding this diet so that you understand it a little better.

So what are some recommended foods?

Eggs, lean proteins, low carb vegetables, limited fruit, zero calorie beverages, and grapefruit are the recommended foods. It's best to avoid pastas, most breads, and other starches such as rice and potatoes. If you need bread, then try a slice of meal bread, which is a bread that's made of nuts and seeds such as rye.

Do I need to exercise with this diet?

Exercise isn't actually required for this diet plan. Though, you'll get better results if you do exercise lightly. Just keep in mind that you won't be able to use strenuous exercise since you're using a low carb and low calorie diet. If you want to exercise when you're on the hardboiled egg diet, try light exercise such as speed walking on a treadmill, light biking, or even just aerobics to stay in shape and help to trim down. Small bursts of exercise are also found to be more effective on this diet than long sessions. Aim for fifteen to twenty minutes once or twice a day.

Is the hardboiled egg diet considered to be expensive?

Since the cost of eggs is reasonable and considered affordable, this is considered to be an inexpensive diet. The only increase in your budget will come from the lean proteins and fresh vegetables if you aren't already budgeting these in. it is also best to buy high quality eggs since they'll be more nutrient dense. If you want to go above and beyond, then you may even want to buy duck eggs! This is easier to do if you live in a rural area, but you can usually find duck eggs in urban areas too. Just check your local classifieds, and be prepared to spend more.

Can you consume any fats on this diet?

You can have butter in this diet, coconut oil, and some mayonnaise. It's best to get the sugar free or even homemade mayonnaise. If you're opting for butter, then grass fed would be best.

Can I have any sweetener?

You want to keep your sweeteners, but you can have up to three servings of sweetener each and every day if you don't drink diet soda, then you can use it for something else. Remember that you should count your fruit as one serving since it does have a natural sugar in it which can decrease your weight loss if eaten in excess. Always have fruit or anything sweet in moderation. You'll want to cut out the sweetener in recipes if possible as well.

Will I suffer from constipation?

If you have a tablespoon of fat per egg you eat, then you likely won't get constipated. Though, if you don't, then you will have to deal with this you can also increase your intake of coconut oil or use fiber to get things moving if you feel it's necessary. Alternatively, you can also add more greens in your diet if you're having a hard time staying full or having bowel movements, since spinach, mustard greens, lettuce, and other vegetables are a large source of dietary fiber.

Will I suffer from digestive issues on this diet?

Not, this shouldn't be the case. You shouldn't have any digestive distress if you're using coconut oil, but o may suffer from flu like symptoms for a few days. Just wait it out, and it'll eventually go away. This is your body trying to adjust to the new diet that you're giving it, especially if you aren't used to a low carb diet.

Will I gain the weight back?

You will not gain the weight back if you go to a low carb diet once you've finished losing the amount of weight you wanted with the hardboiled egg diet. However, if you go back to the Standard American Diet, then you're likely to gain the weight back because of the increased carbs. You'll also want to have a transition period where you wean yourself off of the diet.

Chapter 3: How to Boil an Egg

If you make the perfect hardboiled egg every time, then feel free to skip ahead. If not, here's the basics to the hardboiled egg diet, actually boiling your eggs to perfection. If you can't boil an egg properly, then you'll find many of these recipes harder than necessary, and a properly boiled egg simply tastes better. Once you get the hang of the process, boiling an egg perfectly every time will become second nature.

Step 1: Get Your Eggs Started

You'll want to start with twelve eggs, and then get out a saucepan or pot. Put your eggs in first, and then cover them with cold water. If you put your eggs in second, they might crack while they float to the bottom. Keep in mind that older eggs are easier to peel, so it's okay if you've had them in the fridge or a few weeks! So long as they aren't bad, you'll be able to boil them just fine.

Step 2: Start the Boil

You'll want to put your pan over high heat, and bring your water to a boil. Your water should just come to a boil, but you shouldn't keep it at a boil. Remove the pan from heat. If the eggs stay at high heat or too long, then your yolks will turn green. You don't want to actually boil your eggs at all. The eggs will cook in water that aren't boiling.

Step 3: Let Your Eggs Sit

Your eggs should be allowed to stand in your water for about fourteen to seventeen minutes. How long exactly will depend on how big your eggs are and just how much you want them cooked. For small to medium eggs, only keep them in there for fourteen minutes. For large to extra-large eggs, let them stand for seventeen minutes.

Step 4: Use an Ice Bath

The ice water will cool your eggs down and prevent the yolks from turning green. It's also easier to peel your eggs. Start by draining off your eggs, and then submerge them in an ice water bath. You shouldn't let them stay submerged for more than an hour, but most people only need ten minutes before they can either store them or peel them.

Chapter 4: Recipes to Get You Started

Here are some recipes to get you started on your journey. In this chapter you'll find egg recipes that can be used for various parts of the day, and the variety is meant to liven up the otherwise boring routine. Just because you need to eat hardboiled eggs at least two times a day doesn't mean they have to be plain. Just keep in mind that for recipes that use bacon, you should use them sparingly. Substitute the bacon for turkey bacon if at all possible too.

Eggs on a Bed

Serves: 2

Time: 10 Minutes

Ingredients:

- 2 Hard Boiled Eggs
- Sea Salt to Taste
- Coconut Oil
- Avocado, Sliced
- Spinach to Taste
- 1 Slice Whole Wheat Bread

Directions:

1. Peel and slice your eggs, and season with them with salt before serving. Place them on the plate next to your bread and sliced avocado.
2. Heat up your oil in the skillet with a handful of spinach, allowing it to wilt before placing it on the plate to serve.
3. Serve warm.

Onion Skin Eggs

Serves: 5

Time: 50 Minutes

Ingredients:

- 5 Eggs
- 2 Yellow Onions
- 2 Red Onions

Directions:

1. Start by removing the colored skins rom outside of your red and yellow onion. Save the inside for later, and then take out a cheesecloth. You'll want to cut it in five inch squares, placing a couple of pieces of onion skin into each piece. Set an egg on top, and then gather the cheesecloth around the egg so that the egg is covered in onion skin. Secure the cheesecloth with a rubber band.

2. Get out a pot of cold water, and then place your wrapped eggs inside. Bring it to a boil, and then remove it from heat. Allow it to stand in the water for teen to fifteen minutes.
3. Rinse your eggs under cold water, snipping off the rubber bands.
4. Prepare your eggs like you normally would.

Salmon Deviled Eggs

Serves: 5

Time: 40 Minutes

Ingredients:

- ¼ Clove Garlic, Pressed
- 1 Tablespoon Vegetable Oil
- 2 Teaspoons Vegetable Oil
- Sea Salt & Black Pepper to Taste
- 1 ¼ Teaspoons Red Wine Vinegar
- 3 Eggs Yolks, Room Temperature
- 2-3 Eggs
- ¼ Shallot, Minced
- 6 Ounces Salmon, Canned, Drained & Flakes

Directions:

1. You'll need to start by making your mayonnaise, so beat your egg yolks in a bowl with a hand blender. Slowly

blend in your oil a teaspoon at a time, making sure to mix constantly. Your homemade mayonnaise should be a little thicker than store bought mayonnaise.

2. Piece your garlic clove, and then stir it around in the mixture. It should release its juices, and then remove it. Season the mixture with salt and pepper.

3. Mix in your red wine vinegar a teaspoon at a time, making sure to go slow.

4. Put your eggs in a pot, and boil them like you normally would. Submerge them in your ice bath, and when you're ready to peel them cut them in half lengthwise. Remove the yolks, placing them in another bowl. Put your egg whites on a serving dish.

5. Add your shallots, salmon and a half a cup of

mayonnaise to your yolks. Season with salt and pepper, blending well. If your mixture seems to dry, then add in more mayonnaise as needed.

6. Spoon the mixture into your egg whites, and serve chilled.

Egg & Asparagus Salad

Serves: 4

Time: 30 Minutes

Ingredients:

- 3 Tablespoons Coconut Oil
- 2 Cloves Garlic, Chopped
- 1 lb. Asparagus, Chopped into 3 Inch Pieces
- ½ Teaspoon Sea Salt, Fine
- 4 Hardboiled Eggs, Peeled & Quartered
- Black Pepper to Taste
- 1 Lemon, Sliced

Directions:

1. Start by heating up your oil in a skillet using medium heat, and then stir in your garlic, cooking until fragrant. This should take about a minute.
2. Add in your asparagus, stirring occasionally as you

season with salt. Cook until its tender, which should take about three to five minutes. Allow it to cool in the skillet once you've turned off the heat.

3. Stir in your egg quarters, and then season with pepper and garnish with your lemon slices.

Spinach & Egg Salad

Serves: 7

Time: 40 Minutes

Ingredients:

- ½ Cup White Sugar
- 1 Cup Coconut or Vegetable Oil
- ½ Cup White Vinegar
- 2 Tablespoons Worcestershire Sauce
- 1/3 Cup Ketchup
- 1 Onion, Small & Chopped
- 5 Slices Bacon
- 3 Eggs
- 1 lb. Spinach, Fresh & Torn
- 4 Ounces Water Chestnuts, Sliced & Drained

Directions:

1. IN a blender process your sugar, oil, Worcestershire sauce, vinegar, ketchup and

onion until smooth. Set this mixture to the side.

2. Put your bacon in a skillet, cooking using medium-high heat. It should brown, and then drain it. Crumble your bacon before setting it to the side.

3. Put your eggs in a saucepan, covering them with cold water. Boil like you normally would, and then peel and chop them.

4. In a bowl, toss your spinach, water chestnuts, eggs and bacon together. Serve with a dressing of your choice.

Creamed Eggs

Serves: 4

Time: 30 Minutes

Ingredients:

- 8 Hardboiled Eggs
- 2 Tablespoons Butter, Grass Fed
- 2 Tablespoons All Purpose Flour
- 1 Cup Whole Milk
- ¼ Cup Parmesan Cheese, Grated
- Sea Salt & Black Pepper to Taste

Directions:

1. Melt your butter in a saucepan over medium heat, whisking in your flour. Once blended, slowly stir in your milk. Make sure to stir constantly, and then cook

until it's thickened. Stir in your cheese.
2. Chop your boiled eggs, and then pour your sauce over them before serving.

Teriyaki Eggs

Serves: 6

Time: 6 Hours 33 Minutes

Ingredients:

- 6 Hardboiled Eggs
- ½ Cup Water
- ½ Cup Soy Sauce
- 6 Tablespoons White Sugar
- 1 Tablespoon Onion, Dried & Minced
- ½ Teaspoon Sesame Oil

Directions:

1. Get out a quart size mason jar and peel your eggs, placing them in the jar.
2. Combine your water, sugar, and soy sauce together. Mix in your sesame oil and minced onion, and then cook the mixture over medium heat in a saucepan. Stir and cook until your sugar is

dissolved, which should take about three to five minutes.

3. Pour the mixture over your eggs, and then refrigerate for at least six hours before serving. Remember that these will now count as a serving of sweetener.

Polished Eggs

Serves: 4

Time: 35 Minutes

Ingredients:

- 4 Hardboiled Eggs
- 4 Tablespoons Soy Sauce
- 2 Tablespoons Brown Sugar
- 4 Cloves Garlic, Crushed
- 2 Tablespoons Vegetable Oil

Directions:

1. When you peel your eggs, score the spirals into the whites of your egg.
2. Take out a saucepan, heating up your oil. Add in your garlic, cooking over medium heat. It should begin to brown, and then stir in your sugar and soy sauce, taking your pan from heat.
3. Put your eggs in your sauce, turning them to coat. When

they're nice and dark,
remove them from the sauce
to serve. The sauce should
be thick and syrupy.
Remember that this would be
considered a serving of
sweetener.

Buffalo Ranch Deviled Eggs

Serves: 4

Time: 45 Minutes

Ingredients:

- 3/8 Stalk Celery
- Cayenne Pepper to Taste
- 2 Cups Hot Buffalo Wing Sauce
- 1 Tablespoon + 1 Teaspoon Ranch Salad Dressing
- 2 Hardboiled Eggs

Directions:

1. Once you've peeled your eggs cut them in half lengthwise, and then put your yolks in a bowl.
2. Mash your yolks before stirring in our buffalo sauce and your ranch stir until smooth, spooning the mixture back into your egg whites.

3. Serve sprinkled with cayenne pepper, and chop your celery. Either serve your celery on the side or diced on the top of your deviled eggs.

Simple Salad

Serves: 4

Time: 30 Minutes

Ingredients:

- 1 Tablespoon Corn Oil
- 1 Tablespoon Red Wine Vinegar
- Sea Salt & Black Pepper to taste
- 1 Carrot, shredded
- 1 Tomato, Sliced
- ½ Head Lettuce, Chopped
- 2 Chicken Breasts, Sliced & Cooked
- 2 Hardboiled Eggs

Directions:

1. Start by cooking your bacon, and then drain and crumble it. Set your bacon to the side.
2. Peel and chop your eggs.
3. Put your lettuce in a salad bowl, adding in your tomato

and carrot. Sprinkle with eggs and bacon, and then toss until mixed.

4. Drizzle your oil and vinegar over your salad, sprinkling with salt and pepper before serving.

Chesapeake Deviled Eggs

Serves: 5

Time: 55 Minutes

Ingredients:

- 3 Hardboiled Eggs
- ½ Teaspoon Dry Mustard
- 1 ½ Ounces Blue Crab Meat, Cooked
- ¾ Teaspoon Coconut Oil
- ½ Teaspoon Old Bay Seasoning
- 3 Tablespoons + 1 Teaspoon Water

Directions:

1. Peel and cut your eggs lengthwise, and then put your yolks in a bowl. Mash your yolks before stirring in your Old Bay, oil, crab meat, and dry mustard. Beat the mixture with an electric mixture on low speed until smooth. Add your water

gradually as needed until you get the desired consistency.

2. Put your egg whites on a serving platter, spooning your yolk mixture into them. Sprinkle with more seafood seasoning if desired.

Pickled Eggs

Serves: 6

Time: 1 Day 12 Minutes

Ingredients:

- 3 Hardboiled Eggs
- 15 Ounces Pickled Beets, Canned
- 1 Tablespoon Red Onion, Sliced

Directions:

1. Peel your eggs before placing them in a wide mouthed jar. Pour your picked beets and juice over them, and then add in your onions.
2. Put the lid on the jar, and then place it in the fridge for at least twenty-four hours. Two days will result in a stronger taste. You'll need to stir your jar at least once to make sure that your eggs become evenly covered

3. Slice your eggs before serving.

Avocado Egg Salad

Serves: 3

Time: 10 Minutes

Ingredients:

- 1 Avocado, Peeled, Pitted & Mashed
- 3 Hard Boiled Eggs, Peeled & Chopped
- Sea Salt to Taste
- 1 Tablespoon Celery, Chopped
- 1 Tablespoon Onion, Chopped
- 1 Tablespoon Sweet Pickle Relish

Directions:

1. Mix all ingredients together before serving.

Cauliflower Egg Salad

Serves: 6

Time: 2 Hours 35 Minutes

Ingredients:

- 3 Hard Boiled Eggs, Chopped
- 1 Head Cauliflower, Trimmed into Florets
- ¾ Cup Mayonnaise, Sugar Free
- 1 Tablespoon Mustard
- Ground Black Pepper to Taste
- 1 Onion, Chopped
- ¼ Cup Dill Pickles, Chopped
- ¾ Cup Green Peas, Frozen & Thawed

Directions:

1. Put your cauliflower in a saucepan before covering it with water, bringing the pan to a boil. Cook until your cauliflower is tender, and then drain. It should take

about ten minutes. Allow your cauliflower to cool.

2. In a bowl whisk your mayonnaise, mustard, sea salt, and pepper together.

3. Add your onions, peas, eggs, dill pickles, cauliflower and dressing together, stirring until everything is coated.

4. Refrigerate for two to twenty-four hours before serving. The longer you leave it to chill the stronger the flavor.

Egg Guacamole

Serves: 1

Time: 23 Minutes

Ingredients:

- 1 Avocado
- 1 Hardboiled Egg

Directions:

1. Peel your egg and then mash it with the avocado, making sure it's well combined.

Tuna Salad

Serves: 4

Time: 15 Minutes

Ingredients:

- French Dressing to taste
- 1 Head Iceberg Lettuce, Torn
- 1 Cucumber, Peeled & Diced
- 5 Ounces Tuna, Canned & Drained
- 15 Ounces Chickpeas, Drained
- 2 Hardboiled Eggs

Directions:

1. Mix your tuna, chickpeas, hardboiled egg, lettuce and cucumber together in a bowl.
2. Toss well before adding in your French dressing, and serve immediately.

Egg Kulambu

Serves: 8

Time: 1 Hour

Ingredients:

- 8 Hardboiled Eggs
- ½ Teaspoon Black Peppercorns, Whole
- ½ Teaspoon Cumin Seeds
- ½ Teaspoon Fennel Seeds
- 3 Tablespoons Coconut Oil
- ½ Teaspoon Ground Turmeric
- 1 Onion, Large & Sliced Thin
- 2 Tomatoes, Chopped
- 6 Cloves Garlic, Minced
- 1 Tablespoon Ginger Root, Fresh & Minced
- 1 Teaspoon Ground Red Pepper
- 11/2 Teaspoon Ground Coriander
- ¼ Cup Coconut, Shredded
- ¼ Cup Palm Sugar

- ¼ Cup Cilantro Leaves, Fresh & Chopped
- 1 Cup Water
- ½ Teaspoon Tamarind Paste
- Sea Salt to Taste

Directions:

1. Peel your eggs and cut four slits into each one.
2. Roast your cumin, peppercorns, and fennel seeds over medium heat in a skillet. Cook until fragrant, and then grind them into a powder before setting them to the side.
3. Heat oil in a large skillet, stirring in your oil and turmeric. Fry your eggs in the oil, making sure to fry all the sides. It should take about two minutes, and then set them to the side.
4. Cook your onions in the oil until they turn golden brown, adding in your garlic, ginger and tomatoes continue to

cook until your tomatoes are sot, and then stir in your red pepper, seed mixture, coriander and onion. Cook for another one to two minutes.

5. Pour your water into the skillet, adding in your palm sugar, tamarind, sea salt and coconut. Return the mixture to a boil, and then cook until it starts to thicken. This should take about five minutes.

6. Reduce the heat to medium-low, and add in your eggs. Allow it to simmer for ten minutes. If your sauce is too thick then thin it out with water.

7. Garnish with your cilantro before serving warm.

Wasabi Deviled Eggs

Serves: 5

Time: 50 Minutes

Ingredients:

- 3 Hardboiled Eggs
- 1 Tablespoon + 2 Teaspoons Mayonnaise
- 2 ¾ Teaspoons Green Onions, Minced
- ½ Teaspoon Rice Wine Vinegar
- ½ Teaspoon Wasabi Paste
- 5 Pickled Ginger Slices
- 2 Tablespoons + 1 ½ Teaspoons Fresh Pea Shoots
- Sea Salt to Taste

Directions:

1. Cut your eggs lengthwise after peeling them, putting your egg yolks in a bowl. Mash your yolks until they become smooth, adding in your green onions, rice wine

vinegar, mayonnaise, and wasabi paste. Season with sea salt before continuing.

2. Arrange your egg whites halves on a platter before spooning your yolk mixture into the egg whites. Garnish with pickled ginger and pea shoots before serving.

Egg Curry

Serves: 2

Time: 35 Minutes

Ingredients:

- 2 Tablespoons Coconut Oil
- 1 Teaspoon Garlic Paste
- 1 Onion, Sliced
- ½ Teaspoon Ginger Paste
- 1 Tablespoon Ground Coriander
- 1 Teaspoon Ground Cumin
- ½ Teaspoon Chile Powder
- ½ Teaspoon Ground Turmeric
- ¼ Cup Tomato Puree
- ¼ Teaspoon Black Pepper
- 1 ¼ Cups Water
- 1 Tablespoon Vinegar
- 4 Hardboiled Eggs, Halved
- Sea Salt to Taste

Directions:

1. Heat your oil over medium heat in a large pot, adding in

your onion. Cook until it's browned, which should take about five minutes.

2. Add in your ginger and garlic paste, mixing in your Chile powder, coriander, turmeric, cumin, and black pepper. Cook until it's fragrant, which should take about a minute.

3. Add in your tomato puree, cooking until it thickens. It should take about four minutes.

4. Pour your water into a pot, bringing the mixture to a boil. Add in your sea salt and vinegar, slipping your eggs into the pot. Cook for about five more minutes before serving.

Bacon Jalapeno Deviled Eggs

Serves: 24

Time: 35 Minutes

Ingredients:

- 12 Hardboiled Eggs
- 1/3 Cup Mayonnaise, Sugar Free
- ½ Lemon, juiced
- ¼ Cup Bacon, Chopped & Cooked
- 2 Tablespoons Cheddar, Shredded
- 2 Teaspoons Jalapeno, Chopped
- 1 ½ Tablespoons Yellow Mustard
- Sea Salt & Black Pepper to Taste

Directions:

1. Peel your eggs before cutting them in half, and then place your yolks in a bowl. Put your egg whites on a plate

2. Use a fork to mash your yolks, adding in your lemon juice, mayonnaise, mustard, jalapeno, cheddar and bacon. Season with salt and pepper before mixing again.
3. Spoon the mixture back into your egg whites.

Dill Pickle Deviled Eggs

Serves: 12

Time: 30 Minutes

Ingredients:

- 6 Hardboiled Eggs
- ¼ Cup Mayonnaise, Sugar Free
- 2 Tablespoons Dill Pickles, Minced
- 1 Teaspoon Dijon Mustard
- 1 Teaspoon Pickle Juice
- Old Bay Seasoning to Taste
- Sea Salt & Black Pepper to Taste
- Cornichons, Sliced for Garnish

Directions:

1. Peel and halve your eggs lengthwise, and scoop the yolks out to place them in a bowl.
2. Mash your egg yolks, adding in your pickle juice, mustard,

and mayonnaise and then stir in your pickles. Season with salt and pepper.

3. Scoop the mixture back into your egg whites, and then sprinkle with your Old Bay seasoning and garnish with cornichons

Special Bacon Blue Eggs

Serves: 18

Time: 2 Hours

Ingredients:

- ½ Cup Mayonnaise, Sugar Free
- Sea Salt & Black Pepper to Taste
- Garlic Powder to Taste
- 18 Large Hardboiled Eggs
- 2 Heads Garlic
- 10 Asparagus Spears, Trimmed
- 10 Slices Bacon, Thick Cut (Optional)
- ¼ Cup Plain Greek Yogurt
- 1 ½ Tablespoons Dijon mustard
- Sea Salt & Black Pepper to Taste
- ½ Teaspoon Smoked Paprika
- 2 Ounces Blue Cheese, Crumbled
- 2 Tablespoons Fresh Chives

Directions:

1. Start by heating your oven to 350, and then slice the heads off of your garlic, drizzling them with olive oil.
2. Wrap them tightly with foil, placing them in the oven allow them to roast for forty-five to sixty minutes. Remove your garlic once the time is up, and unwrap it. They'll be golden and caramel-y. Allow it to cool for to the touch
3. Place a skillet over medium-low heat, cooking all of your bacon until crisp. Put your bacon on a paper towel, and only keep about one tablespoon of grease in the skillet. Add in your asparagus to your skillet, seasoning with your salt, pepper and garlic. Allow it to cook until slightly softened, which

should take about five minutes. Turn the heat off.

4. Slice a very small portion of the egg off of the bottom, and then slice the upper half of the egg to reveal the yolk. Scoop out the yolk.

5. In a food processor add in your bacon until they crumble, and then set them to the side.

6. Place your mayonnaise, yogurt, mustard, egg yolks, roasted garlic cloves, pepper and salt in your food processor. Make sure that the skin is removed from your garlic cloves drizzle the remaining grease in until it's smooth and creamy. Scoop the mixture, placing them into your open egg whites. Top the mixture with your bacon, and add some blue cheese crumbs on top. Slice your asparagus in half only if it's needed. And then stick a

stalk in your eggs, standing up.

7. Sprinkle with chives and smoked paprika before serving.

Egg Chaat

Serves: 6

Time: 20 Minutes

Ingredients:

- 3 Hardboiled Eggs
- 1 Tablespoon Ketchup, Sugar Free
- 1 Teaspoon Tomato Chili Paste
- 3 Teaspoons Tamarind Extract
- 1 Teaspoon Cumin, Roasted
- 1 Teaspoon Lemon Juice
- 1 Green Chili
- Sea Salt to Taste
- 1 Spring Onion, Chopped
- 3 Tablespoons Boondi

Directions:

1. Mix your ketchup, chili sauce, lemon juice, green chili, sea salt, roasted cumin, and tamarind extract together

2. Cut your boiled eggs lengthwise, and spread the mixture over them.
3. Sprinkle your spring onion on top as well as your boondi. Serve immediately.

Lean Scotch Eggs

Serves: 6

Time: 45 Minutes

Ingredients:

- 6 Large Hardboiled Eggs
- 2 Large Eggs, Beaten
- 12 Ounces Lean Turkey Breast, Minced
- 1 Teaspoon Mustard Powder, Heaping
- 3 Teaspoons Flat Leaf Parsley, Finely Chopped & Heaping
- 3 Tablespoons Plain Flour
- ½ Teaspoon Curry Powder
- 2 Ounces Mayonnaise, Sugar Free
- 3 ¼ Ounces Breadcrumbs

Directions:

1. Peel your eggs, and then set them to the side.
2. Mix your minced turkey, mustard powder and a

tablespoon of your parsley in a bowl. Season with salt and pepper and mix again.

3. Put your flour in a shallow dish, dusting your eggs in your flour.

4. Divide your minced turkey into six portions, and then flatten them to create a thin round put your eggs in the center, and wrap your meat around the egg.

5. Put your breadcrumbs on a plate, adding in your parsley. Season with salt and pepper and mix well.

6. Dust your meat in the flour, then dip it in your egg mixture, and then roll them in your breadcrumbs until coated.

7. Heat two tablespoons of your oil in a pan, adding in your scotch eggs. Cook over medium heat for about fifteen minutes. They should turn crisp and golden, but

you'll need to turn them often

8. Mix your curry powder and mayonnaise together, and drizzle it over your scotch eggs to serve.

Spicy Egg Salad Celery

Serves: 6

Time: 10 Minutes

Ingredients:

- 8 Hardboiled Eggs, Chopped
- 1 Tablespoons Lemon Juice
- 3 Tablespoons Mayonnaise, Sugar Free
- 2 Tablespoons Chives, Chopped & Divided
- 1 Tablespoon Hot Sauce
- ¾ Teaspoons Paprika, Divided
- Sea Salt & Black Pepper to Taste
- 3 Stalks Celery, Chopped into 4 Inch Pieces

Directions:

1. Start by combining your lemon juice, hot sauce, and a tablespoon of chives, eggs, mayonnaise, and a half a

teaspoon of paprika, sea salt, and black pepper together.

2. Spoon this mixture into your celery, and then sprinkle with the remaining chives and paprika before serving.

Chapter 5: Salad Recipes

Since half of what you need to be eating for the hardboiled egg recipe to work is salad, here are a few salad recipes that you can pair with either a boiled egg or eat all on their own as part of your meal plan. Just remember to use lean cuts of meat if you want this diet to work! The best part is that salads are easy to take on the go, so you won't need to quit your recipe just because you live a busy lifestyle. Eggs will provide you with a healthy amount of protein for lunch while these salads provide you with a portable, nutritious source of vitamins, minerals and nutrients needed to keep your body running smoothly.

Steak Salad

Serves: 4

Time: 35 Minutes

Ingredients:

- 1 Sirloin Steak, Cut into ¾ Inch Pieces
- 1 Teaspoon Garlic & Herb Seasoning Blend
- 6 Cups Romaine Lettuce, Chopped
- 1 Sweet Onion, Cut into Thick Slices
- 6 Hardboiled Eggs, Peeled & Sliced
- 1 Tomato, Sliced

Dressing:

- 1 Tablespoon Garlic & Herb Seasoning Blend
- 1/3 Cup Red Wine Vinegar
- 1 Tablespoon Olive Oil
- 2 Tablespoons Honey, Raw

Directions:

1. Start by combining your dressing ingredients in a bowl, reserving 1/3 cup of your dressing. Brush the remaining dressing on your onion slices
2. Press a tablespoon of seasoning onto your bee steak, putting the steak over a grill, arranging your onions around it grill your onions and steak for seven to eleven minutes, depending on how you like it. Carve your beef into slices.
3. Put your lettuce on a serving platter, topping with your eggs, onions and tomatoes. Drizzle with your /3 cup dressing, and serve immediately.

Cucumber & Tomato Salad

Serves: 4

Time: 10 Minutes

Ingredients:

- 4 Hardboiled Eggs
- 3 Avocados, Peeled, Pitted &Diced
- 1 Red Onion, Small & Thinly Sliced
- ¼ Cup Cilantro, Fresh & Chopped Roughly
- 1 Cucumber, Diced
- 4 Roma Tomatoes, Diced
- 1 Tablespoons Lemon Juice, Fresh
- 2 Tablespoons Olive Oil
- Sea Salt & Black Pepper to Taste

Directions:

1. Peel your hardboiled eggs and chop them.

2. Mix everything together before serving room temperature or chilled.

Cobb Salad

Serves: 2

Time: 10 Minutes

Ingredients:

- 5 Cps Romaine Lettuce, Chopped
- 1 Cup Ham, Diced
- ½ Cup Cherry Tomatoes, Halved
- 1 Avocado, Halved, Seeded, Peeled & Diced
- 2 Hardboiled Eggs, Diced
- ¼ Cup Goat Cheese, Crumbled

Dressing:

- Olive Oil to Taste
- Garlic Powder to Taste
- Sea Salt & Black Pepper to Taste

Directions:

1. Mix all of your dressing ingredients together.

2. Mix all of your salad ingredients together.
3. Drizzle your dressing over your salad before serving.

Cucumber & Dill Salad

Serves: 4

Time: 10 Minutes

Ingredients:

- ¼ Cup Greek Yogurt
- ¼ Cup Red Onion, Sliced
- 2 Cucumbers, Sliced
- 2 Tablespoons Dill, Fresh & Chopped
- 1 Lemon, Juiced & Zested
- Sea Salt & Black Pepper to Taste
- 1 Clove Garlic, Grated

Directions:

1. Mix everything together and enjoy!

Green Bean Salad

Serves: 4

Time: 2 Hours 20 Minutes

Ingredients:

- 2 lbs. Green Beans, Fresh & Trimmed
- ¼ Cup Olive Oil
- 1 Pint Cherry Tomatoes, Halved
- 3 Tablespoons Balsamic Vinegar
- 3 Tablespoons Lemon Juice, Fresh
- ¼ Teaspoon Garlic Powder
- Sea Salt & Black Pepper to Taste
- 4 Ounces Feta Cheese, Crumbed

Directions:

1. Start by boiling a pot of water, adding in a teaspoon of salt. Allow your green beans to become tender,

cooking for five to ten minutes.

2. Once tender, plunge them into an ice water bath and drain them.
3. Pat them dry, and toss them in with your tomatoes.
4. Whisk together your vinegar, salt, garlic, pepper, olive oil and lemon juice together to make your dressing. Pour this mixture over your green beans and tomatoes, stirring to coat.
5. Cover your bowl, placing it in the fridge for up to three hours before serving with feta cheese on top.

Balsamic Beet Salad

Serves: 4

Time: 20 Minutes

Ingredients:

Beets:

- 1 ½ lbs. Beets
- 3 Tablespoons Balsamic Vinegar
- 1 Tablespoon Olive Oil

Salad:

- 6 Cups Arugula
- 2 Ounces Goat Cheese, Crumbled
- 2 Tablespoons Walnuts, Chopped

Directions:

1. Start by removing the greens from your beets and cleaning them. Place them in a saucepan with about an inch of water. Boil your beets for about thirty-five to forty

minutes. They should become tender.

2. Cool them under cold water before removing the skins, and then cut them into quarters once they reach room temperature.

3. Mix about three tablespoons of balsamic vinegar and a tablespoon of oil into a pan, and place it over low heat.

4. Allow the mixture to cool.

5. Divide your arugula onto four plates, placing your beets on top. Sprinkle with goat cheese and walnuts.

6. Drizzle with your dressing mixture before serving.

Massaged Kale Salad

Serves: 6

Time: 10 Minutes

Ingredients:

- 10 Ounces Kale, Raw
- 1/3 Cup Olive Oil
- 4 Cloves Garlic, Minced
- ¼ Cup Lemon Juice, Fresh
- Sea Salt & Black Pepper to Taste

Directions:

1. Place all ingredients into a salad bowl, and massage the kale with your hands for three to four minutes. This will start to soften the kale and bruise it.
2. Serve immediately.

Grilled Romaine Lettuce Salad

Serves: 4

Time: 10 Minutes

Ingredients:

- 3 Tablespoons Olive Oil
- 2 Heads Romaine Lettuce, Cut into 4 Halves
- Sea Sal t& Black Pepper to Taste
- 1 Lemon, Halved
- Feta Cheese, Crumbled

Directions:

1. Turn your grill to medium high, and then brush your lettuce halves with your oil liberally. You need to brush both sides, and sprinkle salt over them.
2. Grill for three minutes with the cut side down, and then flip your lettuce. Grill for two more minutes.
3. Remove your lettuce from the grill, seasoning with salt and pepper before drizzling your olive oil over it.

4. Squeeze your lemon over each half, and then top with feta before serving.

Watermelon & Feta Salad

Serves: 6

Time: 15 Minutes

Ingredients:

- ½ Lime, Sliced
- 2 Tablespoons Olive Oil
- 2 Cups Cucumber, Sliced
- Sea Salt to Taste
- ¼ Cup Red Onion, Sliced Thin
- 1 Cup Feta, Crumbled
- 4 Cups Watermelon, Seedless & Cubed

Directions:

1. Start by placing all ingredients in a bowl.
2. Whisk your olive oil, sea salt and lime juice together.
3. Pour it over the salad, and toss to coat.
4. Serve room temperature or chilled.

Chapter 6: More Vegetable Pairings

Remember that since eggs contain no fiber, you need to pair the hardboiled egg diet with vegetables or it to work. You'll also see this done in the meal plan included in this book. Steaming and grilling your vegetables is best, but you can roast them too! Try these recipes along with one to two hardboiled eggs per serving for the best results.

Roasted Bok Choy

Serves: 3

Time: 15 Minutes

Ingredients:

- 1 Tablespoon Olive Oil
- Black Pepper to Taste
- 1 lb. Bok Choy
- ¾ Tablespoons Sugar
- 2 Tablespoons Soy Sauce, Low Sodium
- ½ Tablespoon Apple Cider Vinegar
- ½ Teaspoon Sesame Oil
- ¼ Teaspoon Sesame Seeds

Directions:

1. Start by heating your oven to 400.
2. Rinse your bok choy and trim the stems off. Slice them, and then quarter them.
3. Prepare your dressing by mixing your sesame seeds, sesame oil, sugar, apple

cider vinegar and soy sauce
together.

4. Mix your olive oil and black
   pepper together, and toss in
   your bok choy. Make sure it's
   coated, and then prepare a
   baking sheet with parchment
   paper. Place your bok choy
   on your baking sheet,
   roasting for eight minutes.
5. Drizzle lightly with sauce
   before serving.

Roasted Cabbage

Serves: 4

Time: 55 Minutes

Ingredients:

- ½ Teaspoon Black Pepper
- 1 Teaspoon Sea Salt, Fine
- 2 Teaspoons fennel Seeds
- 1 Tablespoons Garlic Paste
- 2 Tablespoons Olive Oil
- 1 Head Cabbage
- Parsley to Garnish

Directions:

1. Start by heating your oven to 400 before preparing a baking sheet by lining it with parchment paper.
2. Cut your cabbage into slices that are about one inch thick, and then lay them on your baking sheet. Brush them with half of your fennel, salt, pepper, garlic paste and oil. Flip them over, brushing

down the other side with the other half of your ingredients.

3. Bake your cabbage or twenty minutes before flipping it, and then roast for another twenty minutes. Your cabbage should become crisp around the edges.

4. Serve garnished with parsley.

Grilled Baby Bok Choy

Serves: 2

Time: 20 Minutes

Ingredients:

- 2 Baby Bok Choy
- Olive Oil to Coat
- 1 Lemon, Juiced
- Sea Salt & Black Pepper to Taste

Directions:

1. Heat your grill, and then mix your lemon juice, sea salt, pepper and olive oil together in a bowl. Marinate your bok choy in the mixture.
2. Grill for three to five minutes per side, and use your marinade to keep it from drying out if necessary.
3. Serve warm.

Grilled Asparagus

Serves: 4

Time: 10 Minutes

Ingredients:

- 1 lb. Asparagus, Trimmed
- 2 Tablespoons Olive Oil
- 1 Teaspoon Lemon Juice, Fresh
- Sea Salt & Black Pepper to Taste

Directions:

1. Put your asparagus in a zip top bag, adding in your oil, sea salt, black pepper and lemon juice. Close the bag, and make sure to mix the marinade into the asparagus, and then refrigerate or two hours
2. Turn your girl to medium-high, and then grill your asparagus for five minutes. You'll need to turn every

minute or two to keep them from burning.

3. Remove your asparagus from heat, seasoning with salt and pepper before serving.

Steamed Broccoli

Yields: 4 Cups

Time: 35 Minutes

Ingredients:

- 1 ½ lbs. Broccoli
- Sea Salt & Pepper to Taste

Directions:

1. Start by rinsing your broccoli using cold water, shaking off any excess moisture. Cut the broccoli crowns from the stems, and then cut the broccoli into florets.
2. Put an inch of water in a saucepan before lowering in a steamer basket. Bring the water to a boil using high heat.
3. The broccoli should be in a single layer in the basket, so you may need to do up to three baskets, but you'll want to cover the pan.

Reduce the heat to medium, allowing the water to simmer for seven minutes. The broccoli should be a bright green and tender.

4. Season with salt and pepper before serving.

Sautéed Kale

Serves: 4

Time: 25 Minutes

Ingredients:

- 1 lb. Kale, Chopped
- 2 Tablespoons Olive Oil
- ½ Teaspoon Smoked Paprika
- Crushed Red Pepper to taste
- Sea Salt to Taste
- 1 Onion, Chopped

Directions:

1. Start by bringing a pot of water to a boil, seasoning it with salt. Add in your kale, cooking until it's wilted. This should take about five minutes. Drain your kale before setting it to the side.
2. Heat your oil in a pan over medium heat, adding smoked paprika and crushed red pepper. Add in your chopped onion, and cook for

five minutes. Your onion
should become tender.
3. Serve warm.

Mustard Greens & Onion

Serves: 4

Time: 15 Minutes

Ingredients:

- 1 Onion, Sliced Thin
- 1 ½ lbs. Mustard Greens, Stems Removed, Sliced 1 Inch Crosswise
- 2 Teaspoons Apple Cider Vinegar
- Sea Salt & Black Pepper to Taste
- 1 Tablespoon Olive Oil

Directions:

1. Heat your oil over medium-high heat, adding in your onion. Season with sea salt and black pepper. You'll need to stir frequently, cooking for six to eight minutes. Your onion should turn golden and become tender.

2. Add in your greens, seasoning with salt and pepper. Cook until they're wilted, which should take two to three minutes. Stir in your vinegar, seasoning with your salt and pepper before serving.

Boiled Cabbage

Serves: 6

Time: 40 Minutes

Ingredients:

- Sea Salt & Black Pepper to Taste
- 1 ½ Cups Water
- 1 ½ Tablespoons Olive Oil
- 1 Head Cabbage, Large & Rinsed

Directions:

1. Cut your cabbage up, discarding the outer leaves.
2. Sear your cabbage in a pot over medium heat in your oil. Make sure it's coated, and then add water. Cover, and turn it on low. Cook it for ten minutes until your cabbage is tender.

Chapter 7: Lean Meats to Add In

With the hardboiled egg diet, it's important that you eat lean meats to lose the weight you want. Of course, most people don't understand what lean meats entail. There are a few different options, so in this chapter you'll learn the different types of lean meats you can add into your diet and still shed those pounds.

Skinless Poultry

Skinless is very important if you're hoping for the meat to be lean. This includes more than chicken though. It includes turkey, chicken and Cornish hens. Lean meat is a cut of meat that has less than ten grams of fat per three ounce servings. Poultry can be some of the leanest meats you'll find, and you can cook them a variety of ways.

Lean Beef

You'll get a lot of important nutrients from bee cuts, including vitamin B-12 and iron, which can help to offset the lethargic feeling you get from the hardboiled egg diet. However, it still needs to be eaten in moderation. If you find a beef cut with loin or round in the name, then they're leaner than beef cuts that have the name chuck in the name. Tenderloin, top loin, sirloin tip, and ground round are examples of leaner cuts of beef. Choose the meat that is ninety to ninety-five percent lean if possible, which will keep your fat intake low. You can usually find the percentage printed on the package.

Lamb & Pork

Just like with beef, if you're going for pork or lamb, then look for the word loin in the name. This will have a low fat percentage. Look for pork center loin, pork tenderloin and lamb tenderloin for the best cuts. You'll find that with pork and lamb the fat is usually visible, so you can actually trim it off with a sharp knife before you cook it.

Fish

Fish is packed with lean protein, and your leanest choices are white fish. This includes tilapia, flounder and even most shellfish including lobster. Dark meat fish such as salmon and tuna are also lean since the fat they have are healthy fat, making it perfect for the hardboiled egg diet. Fish oils will help your body to regulate its metabolism, helping you to lose weight quickly. It can also reduce inflammation and regulate your hormones.

Keeping Your Meat Lean

To keep your meat lean, then you'll want to steam, grill, poach, broil or bake it. This will keep the fat content low. You will not want to sauté your meat or fry it often. With the hardboiled egg diet, you'll find that most of the oil you need will be found in your vegetables, so you should add as little as possible to your meat. Only lightly season your meat, using natural herbs. You'll want to try thyme, sage, rosemary or other fresh herbs.

What about Bacon?

Bacon isn't lean, and so you should use it sparingly when you're using the hardboiled egg diet. Of course, you can always use turkey bacon which is at least leaner than traditional pork bacon. Even with turkey bacon, use it sparingly, but bacon grease will help to keep your bowel movements regular so that you won't have to worry about constipation during this diet.

Chapter 8: Lean Meat Recipes

Now that you know what meats to cook, this chapter will cover a few easy recipes to pair with your hardboiled eggs.

Lemon Grilled Salmon

Serves: 2

Time: 15 Minutes

Ingredients:

- 12 Ounces Wild Salmon
- Sea Salt to Taste
- 4 Teaspoons Olive Oil
- 1 Lemon, Fresh

Directions:

1. Start by combining your lemon zest and olive oil together, rubbing it on your salmon.
2. Season your salmon with sea salt, and allow it to sit for two to three minutes.
3. Heat your grill to medium low heat, and then add on your salmon. Grill for four to five minutes with the skin side up, and then flip it over. Cook for another four to five minutes.

4. Remove your salmon from heat, and squeeze your lemon over it before serving.

Easy Baked Chicken

Serves: 4

Time: 20 Minutes

Ingredients:

- ½ Teaspoon Garlic Powder
- ½ Teaspoon Onion Powder
- ½ Teaspoon Chili Powder
- Sea Salt & Black Pepper to Taste
- 2 Tablespoons Olive Oil
- 4 Chicken Breasts, Boneless & Skinless

Directions:

1. Start by heating your oven to 450 degrees, and then pound your chicken until they are of an even thickness.
2. Grease a thirteen by nine inch baking pan with olive oil, and dredge your chicken through it. Place your chicken breasts in the dish.

3. Whisk your sea salt, pepper, onion powder, garlic powder and chili powder together. Sprinkle the seasoning over both sides of your chicken, rubbing it in with your hands.

4. Bake for fifteen to twenty minutes before covering it with foil. Allow it to rest for five to ten minutes before slicing.

Lemon & Basil Pork Chops

Serves: 4

Time: 35 Minutes

Ingredients:

- 4 Pork Loin Chops, Boneless & Cut Thick
- 2 Tablespoons Olive Oil
- 3 Tablespoons Garlic, Minced
- 1 Cup Basil Leaves, Fresh & Minced
- 3 Tablespoons Lemon Juice
- 1 Teaspoon Sea Salt, Fine
- ¾ Teaspoon Black Pepper

Directions:

1. Add your basil, garlic, lemon juice, olive oil, sea salt and pepper together in a bowl before setting it to the side.
2. Spread your mixture over your pork chops, letting them set for twenty minutes.
3. Grill your pork chops for five to six minutes for each side,

and then let it rest for five minutes before serving.

Baked Pork Chop

Serves: 4

Time: 30 Minutes

Ingredients:

- 4 Pork Chops, Bone In
- Cooking Spray as Needed
- Sea Salt & Black Pepper to Taste
- ½ Tablespoon Paprika
- 1 Teaspoon Garlic Powder

Directions:

1. Start by heating your oven to 400 degrees, and then take out a bowl
2. Mix your paprika, garlic powder, sea salt and black pepper together rub the mixture on your pork chops, and then heat an oven safe pan over high heat. Heat it for three minutes and then spray it with cooking spray. Add your pork chops in,

searing them for two minutes per side. Bake or five to ten minutes, and then let rest for five minutes before serving.

Grilled Greek Lemon Chicken

Serves: 4

Time: 2 Hours 15 Minutes

Ingredients:

- 4 Chicken Breasts, Boneless & Skinless Halved
- 1/3 Cup Olive Oil + More for Grilling
- 1 Tablespoon Lemon Zest
- 1/3 Cup Lemon Juice, Fresh
- 2 Teaspoons Oregano, Dried
- 4 Cloves Garlic, Minced
- ½ Teaspoon Rosemary, Dried & Crushed
- ½ Teaspoon Thyme, Dried
- ½ Teaspoon Basil, Dried
- Parsley, Fresh & Chopped for Garnish
- Sea Salt & Black Pepper to Taste

Directions:

1. Pound the thicker parts of your chicken to an even

thickness, and then take out a bowl

2. In your bowl, whisk your lemon zest, lemon juice, garlic, basil, olive oil, oregano, thyme, rosemary and basil. Mix well, and then season with sea salt and black pepper, mixing again.

3. Place your chicken in a resalable bag, pouring your mixture in it. Seal your bag, and then rub your marinade over your chicken, allowing it to marinate for two hours.

4. Heat your girl to medium-high heat, and then brush the grill grates with olive oil.

5. Put your chicken on the grill, and then grill for four minutes per side with the lid closed.

6. Let your chicken rest for five minutes before garnishing with parsley or slicing to serve with a salad.

Grilled Blackened Tuna

Serves: 2

Time: 15 Minutes

Ingredients:

- 2 Tuna Steaks
- 2 Tablespoons Paprika
- 1 Tablespoon Oregano
- 1 Tablespoon Thyme
- ½ Teaspoon Garlic Powder
- ½ Teaspoon Onion Powder
- Sea Salt & Black Pepper to Taste
- 1 Teaspoon Cayenne Pepper

Directions:

1. Start by heating your grill to high, and then spray your fish with cooking spray. Season the top with your spice blend.
2. Put your sprayed side down on the grill, and then close the lid. Cook for one to two

minutes, and then spray the other side and flip. Cook for another one to two minutes. The middle should still be rare when you serve your fish warm.

Cajun Baked Salmon

Serves: 4

Time: 20 Minutes

Ingredients:

- 2 Tablespoons Paprika
- 1 Tablespoon Cayenne Pepper
- 1 Tablespoon Onion Powder
- ½ Teaspoon White Pepper
- 2 Teaspoons Sea Salt, Fine
- ½ Teaspoon Black Pepper
- 1 Teaspoon Thyme, Dried
- 1 Teaspoon Basil, Dried
- 1 Teaspoon Oregano, Dried
- 4 Salmon Fillets, Boneless
- ¼ Cup Butter, Unsalted & Melted

Directions:

1. Start by heating your oven to 450, and then get out a small bowl.
2. Mix all of your dry ingredients into the bowl.

3. Prepare a baking sheet by covering it in foil, which should keep the skin from the fillets rom sticking.

4. Brush your salmon down with your butter, sprinkling the seasoning mixture over it. Gently rub the seasoning mixture in, and then bake for fifteen to seventeen minutes. Your salmon should become flaky.

Broiled Flounder with Lemon Butter

Serves: 2

Time: 10 Minutes

Ingredients:

- 2 Flounder Fillets
- 2 Tablespoons Olive Oil
- 2 Tablespoons Whole Butter
- ½ Teaspoon Chili Flakes
- 1 Lemon
- Sea Salt & Black Pepper to Taste

Directions:

1. Start by heating up your broiler, and then get out a glass baking dish.
2. Add your lemon juice, chili flakes, olive oil and butter in your dish, and then place it in the oven for a minute. This should melt your butter, and then mix.

3. Season your fish with sea salt and black pepper, and then dredge your fish through the melted butter. Place your flounder under your broiler for six to eight minutes.
4. Serve warm.

Rosemary & Garlic Grilled Lamb

Serves: 4

Time: 1 Hour 20 Minutes

Ingredients:

- 1 Lemon, Zested
- 2 lbs. Lamb Loin
- 4 Cloves Garlic, Minced
- 1 Tablespoon Rosemary, Fresh & Chopped
- ¼ Cup Olive Oil
- Sea Salt & Black Pepper to Taste

Directions:

1. Start by combining your garlic, sea salt, pepper, olive oil, and rosemary and lemon zest together.
2. Pour this marinade over your lamb loin, and then flip them over. You want them to be covered completely, and marinate them for an hour.

3. Heat your grill to medium high heat, searing your lamb loin on each side. Lower the heat to medium, and cook for five to six minutes.
4. Allow it to cool before serving.

Grilled Sirloin

Serves: 2

Time: 15 Minutes

Ingredients:

- 2 Sirloin Steaks
- 1 Teaspoon Onion Powder
- 1 Teaspoon Garlic Powder
- 1 Teaspoon Paprika
- 1 Teaspoon Chili Powder
- 1 Teaspoon Brown Sugar
- 1 Tablespoon Black Pepper
- 1 Tablespoon Sea Salt, Fine

Directions:

1. Mix all of your seasonings together, and rub it into your steak. Allow it to stand for five minutes.
2. Prepare your grill by turning it to medium-high heat, and then cook your steak for three to five minutes per side.

3. Allow to rest for two to three minutes before serving.

Lemon Pepper Tilapia

Serves: 2

Time: 10 Minutes

Ingredients:

- 2 Tilapia Fillets
- Olive Oil Spray as Needed
- 1 Teaspoon Lemon Pepper Seasoning

Directions:

1. Get out enough foil to cover each tilapia fillet, and then heat up your grill.
2. Spray your foil with your olive oil, and then put your tilapia on each piece of foil.
3. Season your fillets with lemon pepper seasoning, and then old the foil over your tilapia to create a packet.
4. Grill for eight minutes, and then serve warm.

Chapter 9: Different Types of Eggs

Wait! Before going any further, you're going to want to figure out what type of egg you want to use. All of the recipes in the previous chapter can be done with normal, white eggs you get from the grocery store, but not every egg is made the same.

Brown Eggs vs. White Eggs

You've probably already seen that brown eggs are much more expensive than white eggs. Though, price isn't an indication of how healthy an egg actually is. The difference between brown and white eggs is the difference between the chickens laying them. Chickens with white earlobes will lay white eggs chickens with brown or red earlobes will lay brown eggs.

Of course, not each and every chicken follows these rules. There are even blue and green eggs out there.

Urocyanin is a pigment that results in blue eggs, and porphyrins is a pigment that results in brown eggs. Contrary to popular belief, color isn't linked to the nutritional value of your eggs. Brown eggs are actually more expensive than white eggs because they come from larger hens, which are larger to feed and more expensive to raise. This means that white eggs are a more economic choice. Depending on who you ask, people will swear that the taste is different. Truthfully, you'd need to try for yourself to see what you think.

Duck Eggs vs. Chicken Eggs

Let's take a quick look at the nutritional difference. For the sake of reference, we're going to look at a large chicken egg which is about fifty grams and a duck egg which is about seventy grams.

Chicken Egg:

- **Calories:** 71
- **Total Fat:** 5 Grams
- **Cholesterol:** 211 mg
- **Carbs:** 0 Grams
- **Sodium:** 70 mg
- **Protein:** 6 Grams

Duck Eggs

- **Calories:** 130
- **Fat:** 10 Grams
- **Cholesterol:** 619 Grams
- **Carbs:** 1 Gram
- **Sodium:** 102 mg
- **Protein:** 9 grams

As you can see, the duck egg has more protein, but it also has more calories. Some benefits to eating duck eggs are that they stay fresh longer due to the thicker shell, but this also makes peeling them a little more difficult. Duck eggs also have more omega-3 fatty acids. If you can't eat chicken eggs due to allergies, you're likely able to eat duck eggs though too! People often claim that the nutrition of a duck egg is are superior to that of a chicken egg, but the information is debatable. When it comes down to it with vitamins such as A, D, and E then the duck eggs are the same as the chicken eggs. It all depends on what the bird eats as far as taste goes, many people think that duck eggs are richer and creamier. Some say that it even has a stronger flavor, but once again you'll need to judge or yourself!

Organic

Not all organic labels are equal. You can't just look at the word "organic" and think you know what you're getting. Even with eggs. There are various labels that have been approved by the USDA to describe an organic product there is one hundred percent organic, ninety-five percent organic, and made with organic labels. The made with organic label contains only seventy percent of organic ingredients.

If you have a carton of eggs labeled organic, then you can trust that it's from pesticide, fungicide, herbicide and commercial fertilizer free area. Well, mostly. Remember that organic doesn't meant a hundred percent organic. Though, the term organic actually won't tell you anything about the living condition of your hen or the nutritional value. In short, when you're buying organic eggs, that doesn't mean they have more nutrients. They just won't have trace amounts of pesticides. Since duck eggs have a thicker shell and are larger by nature, you'll want to

let them sit in your hot water for
one to two minutes more.

Omega-3 Enriched

The only difference between these
eggs and normal eggs is that the
hens laying these eggs were fed
omega-3 rich sources. This
includes, and most commonly is,
flaxseeds. These eggs will be
higher in omega-3 fatty acids they
won't have a dramatic effect on
your health, and they can be
unhealthy I the hen was fed poor
quality omega-3 sources.

Vegetarian Fed

You may see this label, and it
means that the hens laying your
eggs were not fed any animal
protein. This may sound healthy,
but it isn't. A hen's natural diet
includes insects and worms,

meaning it isn't naturally vegetarian. You won't notice a significant different between these and white eggs.

Check the Grade of Egg

Grade will determine the freshness of your age, but remember that freshness doesn't make a difference when you're boiling them. So, feel free to go with the cheaper version. An egg that's a few weeks old will actually do better when it comes to peeling!

Chapter 10: One Week Meal Plan

Now that you know what the hardboiled egg diet is, what you need to include, and some recipes to get you started, it's time to actually start. That's where this meal plan will come in handy. If you follow it, you're sure to lose the weight you want! Just stick with it.

Sunday

Breakfast: 2 Boiled Eggs, Small Orange

Lunch: Cobb Salad

Dinner: Cajun Baked Salmon, Steamed Broccoli

Monday

Breakfast: 2 Boiled Eggs, Small Grapefruit

Lunch: 1 Teriyaki Egg, Cucumber & Dill Salad

Dinner: Grilled Sirloin, Sautéed Kale

Tuesday

Breakfast: 2 Boiled Eggs, Small Apple

Lunch: Steak Salad

Dinner: Egg Curry, Roasted Bok Choy

Wednesday

Breakfast: 2 Boiled Eggs, Small Pear

Lunch: 1 Onion Skin Egg, Watermelon & Feta Salad

Dinner: Easy Baked Chicken, Boiled Cabbage

Thursday

Breakfast: Eggs on a Bed

Lunch: Avocado Egg Salad, 1 Slice Meal Bread

Dinner: Lemon & Basil Pork Chops, Grilled Asparagus

Friday

Breakfast: 1 Lean Scotch Egg, Small Apple

Lunch: 2 Wasabi Deviled Eggs, Balsamic Beet Salad

Dinner: Grilled Greek Lemon Chicken, Roasted Cabbage

Saturday

Breakfast: Creamed Eggs, Slice Meal Bread

Lunch: Egg Chaat

Dinner: Grilled Blackened Tuna, Mustard Greens & Onion

Chapter 11: Some Fruit Variety

If you're still looking for some more fruit you can add into the diet, then check out these low carb fruits. They go great with the hardboiled egg diet, and you can swap out any of them in the meal plan. Just remember that you shouldn't have more than one serving of fruit daily if you want to shed those extra pounds on the hardboiled egg diet.

Lemons & Limes

Most people don't want to eat these on their own, but if you do, then they're great to add in! They can help boost your metabolism, but if you don't want to eat them, just add them to your drinking water to get the added benefit.

Blood Oranges

Due to the high level of anthocyanins, blood oranges get their deep red color. This means that they're full of antioxidants too, which can help keep you feeling decent during this diet cleanse. Like most citrus, blood oranges will help to speed your weight loss along too.

Grapefruit

Grapefruits won't raise your blood sugar level after eating, which will help you to lose weight. They can also kick your metabolism into gear. They're also high in vitamin C and low in carbs, which will help you to get through the day and keep from experiencing flu like symptoms on this diet cleanse.

Oranges

Remember to skip the juice when you're trying to lose weight. Oranges, like most citrus, are full of vitamin C. they're also able to provide you with the fiber you need while on the hardboiled egg diet. The citric acid is also known to help boost the metabolism without adding on too many extra calories.

Watermelon

Watermelon is low in carbs, making it a great addition to your hardboiled egg diet. It's also a great way to stay hydrated due to its high water content. You'll also find that watermelon is full of vitamin A while providing very little calories.

Strawberries

Berries are a popular choice for anyone trying to lower their carbs and watch their weight. They're also a great source of vitamin C and potassium. Of course, strawberries are sweeter than other berries, and they should be used sparingly when on the hardboiled egg diet.

Cantaloupe

Melons like cantaloupe and even honeydew go great with tuna salad, and they can be eaten as a snack too. They have very little carbs, and they can help to hydrate you. This makes them a perfect addition to your diet plan without damaging your weight loss goals.

Peaches

Peaches are low in carbs, and they're incredibly sweet. If you're having a hard time sticking to your low carb, hardboiled egg diet plan due to sugar cravings, add in a small peach every few days and it should keep you on track! Just remember that fresh is always best, so never get canned peaches just because they're more convenient.

Chapter 12: Some Extra Tips

It can still be difficult to try out a new diet, and that's where these extra tips come in handy. This will help make your transition into the hardboiled egg diet a little easier, increasing your weight loss results.

Get Your Fiber

You will want to get your fiber from other sources since hard boiled eggs have none. Vegetables are excellent at getting fiber, but chia seeds will help to speed things up too. If you're having a salad, then sprinkle them over it. A teaspoon of chia seeds a day will really help to keep your body functioning like they should. Chia seeds also have omega fats, and five grabs o fiber per tablespoon. If you can't stand chia seeds, then try some fiber supplements.

Keep Hydrated!

Hydrating yourself is incredibly important for weight loss. Not enough people consume the amount of water they need to on a daily basis. It's best to drink six to eight cups of water each and every day. Of course, you will be consuming a fair amount of vegetables, so make sure you aren't crazy with your water intake. Eating cucumbers will also help, and it's a tasty combination too!

Avoid Alcohol & Junk Food

You're going to need to say no to junk food and alcohol for a few weeks if you want this diet to work. it's better to clear out the alcohol and junk food form your home so you aren't tempted, and don't go out with friends if you don't have to. If you do go out, then try not to drink. If you have to drink, then go for straight liquor and skip the cocktails. A gin and tonic has a lot less calories and sweeteners than a margarita.

Get Some Sleep

This may sound like a simple answer, but many people forget to get the sleep they need when trying to lose weight eight hours a night will help you to feel properly rested and keep your body running like a well-oiled machine. Without sleep, you'll find that you're stressed, irritable, and your body won't lose weight nearly as quickly because you'll suffer from slower metabolic function. When you're stressed out, which lack of sleep will cause, your body will cause you to have cravings, bloat, keep weight on, and release higher levels of hormones which will attack muscle mass.

Conclusion

Now you know everything you need to in order to get started with your hardboiled egg diet to get rid of those unwanted pounds. Just make sure that you stick to your first week meal plan, and then develop one that fits your tastes! People often stay on the hardboiled egg diet for as little to one week to as much as six weeks, depending on how much weight they want to lose. Make a plan that works for your weight loss goals, and remember to leave a transition period where you slowly ease yourself back to a healthy, low carb diet so that you don't gain the weight back!

One more thing, if you have enjoyed the book, please leave a review on Amazon. I would really

appreciate it.
Ariel Chandler

Sign Up for Recipes, Tips and Tricks and more at:

HealthyLivingandMore.com

Made in the USA
Middletown, DE
02 May 2018